HEALTHY LIKE CRAZY:

Using the healing power of fasting to burn fat and boost energy.

By Dr. Samantha Colos

TABLE OF CONTENTS:

Introduction

Fasting is the practice of abstaining from food and, in some cases, drink for a specified period of time. It has been a part of human culture and religion for centuries and is approached for various reasons, including spiritual, health, and even scientific purposes.

There are several types of fasting, including:

1. Intermittent Fasting: This involves cycling between periods of eating and fasting. It doesn't prescribe specific foods to eat, but rather when to eat them.

2. Water Fasting: This entails consuming only water for a set period, typically ranging from 24 hours to several days. It's often used for detoxification and cleansing purposes.

3. Juice Fasting: This involves consuming only fruit and vegetable juices along with water. It provides some nutrients while still allowing the digestive system to rest.

4. Religious Fasting: Practiced by many faiths, this involves abstaining from food and sometimes drink for specific periods as a form of spiritual discipline, reflection, and purification.

Fasting can have various benefits, including weight management, improved metabolic health, enhanced mental clarity, and potential spiritual or religious benefits, depending on the individual's goals and intentions.

However, it's crucial to approach fasting with caution and consideration for one's individual health circumstances. Consulting a healthcare professional is recommended, especially for those with underlying medical conditions or if fasting for an extended period.

Understanding the specific type of fast you're interested in, along with its potential benefits and risks, will help you make informed decisions about incorporating fasting into your lifestyle.

CHAPTER 2.
TYPES OF FASTING

- Intermittent Fasting
- Water Fasting
- Juice Fasting
- Religious Fasting Practices

Intermittent fasting is an eating pattern that involves alternating periods of eating with periods of fasting. Unlike traditional diets that focus on specific foods to eat or avoid, intermittent fasting primarily dictates when to eat.

Here are some common methods of intermittent fasting:

1. 16/8 Method: This involves fasting for 16 hours each day and restricting your eating to an 8-hour window. For example, you might eat between 12:00 PM and 8:00 PM and fast from 8:00 PM to 12:00 PM the next day.

2. 5:2 Diet: This approach involves eating normally for five days of the week and significantly reducing calorie intake (around 500–600 calories) on the other two non-consecutive days.

3. Alternate-Day Fasting: This method alternates between days of normal eating and days of very low calorie intake or fasting.

4. Eat-Stop-Eat: This involves a complete fast for 24 hours once or twice a week. For instance, you might eat dinner at 6:00 p.m. and then not eat again until 6:00 p.m. the following day.

5. Warrior Diet: This involves eating small amounts of raw fruits and vegetables during the day and having one large meal in the evening.

Benefits of intermittent fasting may include:

Weight Management: It can help with weight loss by creating a calorie deficit and

improving metabolism.
Metabolic Health: It may improve insulin sensitivity and blood sugar regulation.

Cellular Repair and Autophagy: Fasting triggers a process called autophagy, which is the body's way of cleaning out damaged cells and regenerating new, healthy ones.

Brain Health: Some studies suggest that intermittent fasting may support brain function and reduce the risk of neurodegenerative diseases.

However, it's important to note that intermittent fasting is not suitable for everyone. People with certain medical conditions, pregnant or breastfeeding individuals, and those with a history of eating disorders should consult a healthcare professional before starting any fasting regimen.

As with any dietary change, it's crucial to prioritize balanced nutrition during eating periods and stay hydrated throughout the fasting period. Listening to your body and making adjustments as needed is key to a safe and sustainable intermittent fasting routine.

Water fasting is a type of fasting where an individual consumes only water and abstains from all food and other beverages for a specified period of time. This form of fasting is considered one of the more intense and restrictive fasting methods.
Here are some key points to understand about water fasting:

1. Sole Consumption of Water: During a water fast, the only intake allowed is water. This means no food, juice, or other beverages, including coffee or tea.

2. Duration: Water fasts can range from a few hours to several days or even weeks. Extended water fasts are typically

supervised by healthcare professionals due to their potential risks.

3. Detoxification and Cleansing: Advocates of water fasting often believe it can help cleanse the body of toxins and support overall health. However, scientific evidence on the benefits of detoxification through water fasting is limited and controversial.

4. Potential Benefits: - Autophagy: Water fasting can trigger a process called autophagy, where the body cleans out damaged cells and regenerates new, healthy ones. Weight Loss: Water fasting creates a significant calorie deficit, leading to rapid weight loss. However, this weight loss is often temporary, and long-term changes in diet and exercise are necessary for sustained results.

5. Risks and Considerations: - Dehydration:Without adequate food intake, dehydration can occur. It's essential to drink

enough water to maintain proper hydration levels.Electrolyte Imbalance: Prolonged fasting can lead to imbalances in essential electrolytes like sodium, potassium, and magnesium, which can be dangerous.Nutritional Deficiencies: Long-term water fasting can lead to nutrient deficiencies, potentially causing serious health issues.Medical Supervision: Extended water fasts should be done under the guidance of a healthcare professional to monitor for potential complications.

6. Who Should Avoid Water Fasting?pregnant or breastfeeding individuals.Those with certain medical conditions, including kidney disease, heart disease, and diabetesIndividuals with a history of eating disorders
Before undertaking a water fast, it's crucial to consult with a healthcare provider or registered dietitian to assess whether it's safe and appropriate for your individual health situation. They can provide guidance

on how to approach fasting in a way that minimizes risks and supports your well-being.

Juice fasting, also known as juice cleansing or detoxing, is a type of fasting where individuals consume only fruit and vegetable juices while abstaining from solid food for a specific period of time. Here are some key points to understand about juice fasting:

1. Sole Consumption of Juices: During a juice fast, the primary intake is freshly squeezed juices made from fruits and vegetables. These juices are typically rich in vitamins, minerals, and antioxidants.

2. Duration: Juice fasts can vary in duration, ranging from a few days to several weeks. It's important to establish a clear timeframe and have a plan for gradually reintroducing solid foods.

3. Detoxification and Cleansing: Advocates of juice fasting often believe it can help the body eliminate toxins, support digestion, and promote overall health. However, scientific evidence on the benefits of detoxification through juice fasting is limited and debated.

4. Variety of Juices: A variety of fruits and vegetables can be used to make juices, allowing for a diverse nutrient intake. Common ingredients include leafy greens, citrus fruits, carrots, beets, and more.

5. Potential Benefits:
Nutrient Intake: Fresh juices provide a concentrated source of essential vitamins, minerals, and antioxidants.
Hydration: Juices contribute to hydration, which is vital for overall health and bodily functions.
Digestive Rest: With no solid food to digest, the digestive system gets a break, potentially allowing for rest and rejuvenation.

6. Risks and Considerations:
Nutrient Deficiencies: Juices lack certain nutrients like fiber and protein, which are essential for overall health.
Caloric Intake: While juices are nutritious, they can be low in calories. Prolonged juice fasting may lead to inadequate energy levels.
Blood Sugar Levels: Fruit juices can cause rapid spikes in blood sugar levels due to their natural sugars. This can be a concern for individuals with diabetes or insulin resistance.

7. Who should avoid juice fasting?
pregnant or breastfeeding individuals.
Those with certain medical conditions, including diabetes, kidney disease, and certain gastrointestinal disorders
Individuals with a history of eating disorders
 Before undertaking a juice fast, it's crucial to consult with a healthcare provider or registered dietitian. They can provide

guidance on how to approach juice fasting in a way that minimizes risks and supports your well-being. Additionally, if you experience any adverse effects during the fast, it's important to seek medical attention promptly.

Religious fasting practices are observed by various faith traditions around the world as a form of spiritual discipline, purification, and a means of drawing closer to the divine. These practices often have deep cultural and historical significance. Here are some examples of religious fasting practices from different faiths:

1. Islamic Fasting (Sawm) (Islam):
Ramadan: Muslims observe fasting from dawn to sunset during the month of Ramadan, abstaining from food, drink, smoking, and other physical needs. It's a time of increased devotion, reflection, and community.

2. Lenten Fast (Christianity):
Lent: Christians, particularly in the Catholic and Orthodox traditions, observe a 40-day fast leading up to Easter. This involves various forms of abstinence, including limiting certain foods or meals.

3. Yom Kippur (Judaism):
Known as the Day of Atonement, Yom Kippur involves a 25-hour fast, starting before sunset and ending after nightfall the next day. It's a time of repentance, reflection, and prayer.

4. Ashura (Islam):
This is a day of fasting observed on the 10th day of Muharram, the first month of the Islamic lunar calendar. It has both historical and religious significance in Islamic tradition.

5. Bahai Fasting (Baha'i Faith):
Baha'is observe a 19-day fast from sunrise to sunset during the month of Ala (March 2 to March 21), abstaining from food and drink.

It's a period of spiritual reflection and renewal.

6. Karva Chauth (Hinduism):
Married Hindu women fast from sunrise to moonrise for the well-being and longevity of their husbands. The fast is observed on the fourth day after the full moon in the Hindu month of Kartika.

7. Tisha B'Av (Judaism):
This is a day of mourning and fasting that commemorates various tragedies in Jewish history, including the destruction of the First and Second Temples in Jerusalem.

8. Ritualistic Fasting (Various Indigenous Religions):
Many indigenous cultures have their own fasting traditions as part of rituals or ceremonies, which often serve spiritual, social, or cultural purposes.

These are just a few examples, and there are numerous other religious fasting practices observed around the world. Each practice is deeply meaningful within its respective faith tradition and is often accompanied by specific rituals, prayers, and reflections. It's important to approach these practices with respect and an understanding of their cultural and religious significance.

CHAPTER 3
PREPARING FOR A FAST

- Mental and Emotional Preparation
- Physical Preparations
- Setting Realistic Goals

Preparing for a fast involves several important steps to ensure a safe and successful experience. Here's a guide on how to prepare:

1. Mental and Emotional Preparation:
Set clear intentions: define why you're fasting and what you hope to achieve.
Educate yourself: Learn about the specific type of fast you're undertaking and its potential benefits.
Establish realistic expectations: understand that fasting may be challenging but also empowering.

2. Physical Preparations:

Gradual Transition: If possible, ease into fasting by gradually reducing meal sizes and snacking.
Stay Hydrated: Drink plenty of water leading up to the fast to ensure you're well hydrated.
Nutrient-Rich Meals: Prioritize balanced, nutrient-dense foods in the days leading up to your fast.

3. Plan Your Fasting Period:
Determine the duration and type of fast you'll be undertaking (e.g., intermittent, water, juice).
Choose a Suitable Time: Consider your schedule and pick a time when you can rest and minimize stress.

4. Gather necessary supplies:
Depending on the type of fast, ensure you have any required supplements, juices, or fasting aids.

5. Consult a healthcare professional:

Especially if you have underlying health conditions or are planning an extended fast, seek advice from a healthcare provider.

6. Listen to Your Body:
Pay attention to any signals of discomfort or potential health issues, and be prepared to adjust or end the fast if necessary.

7. Create a Support System:
Let trusted friends or family members know about your fast for moral support and to keep them informed.

8. Mental Preparations:
Practice mindfulness: engage in meditation, deep breathing exercises, or other relaxation techniques.
Manage Stress: Take steps to reduce stress levels in your daily life, as stress can impact your fasting experience.

9. Educate yourself on breaking the fast:

Understand how to gradually reintroduce food post-fast to avoid digestive discomfort.

Remember, fasting is a personal journey, and it's important to approach it with self-awareness and respect for your body's needs. If at any point during your fast you feel unwell or experience concerning symptoms, it's crucial to seek medical attention promptly.

CHAPTER 4

CHOOSING THE RIGHT FAST FOR YOU

- Considering Health Conditions
- Consulting a Healthcare Professional

Choosing the right type of fast is a crucial step in ensuring a positive and beneficial fasting experience. Here are some considerations to help you make an informed decision:

1. Health Considerations:Consider any existing medical conditions or medications you're taking. Certain health conditions may require modifications to fasting plans or may not be compatible with certain types of fasting.

When considering fasting, it's important to take your health into account. Here are some key health considerations to keep in mind:

1. Underlying Medical Conditions:
If you have any existing medical conditions (such as diabetes, heart disease, gastrointestinal disorders, etc.), consult your healthcare provider before starting any fasting regimen. They can provide tailored advice based on your specific situation.

2. Medications:
Some medications may need to be taken with food. Discuss your fasting plans with your healthcare provider to ensure that your medications are compatible with the chosen fasting method.

3. Pregnancy and Breastfeeding:
Pregnant and breastfeeding individuals have specific nutritional needs for themselves and their baby. Fasting may not be appropriate during these periods without guidance from a healthcare professional.

4. Age and Developmental Stage:

Children, adolescents, and older adults may have different nutritional requirements and may need specialized guidance if considering fasting.

5. Nutritional Status:

Consider your current nutritional status. If you are already undernourished, have nutrient deficiencies, or have a history of disordered eating, fasting may not be advisable without proper supervision.

6. Dehydration Risk:

Depending on the type of fast, there may be a risk of dehydration. Ensure you are adequately hydrated before starting any fast, and pay attention to your body's hydration signals throughout.

7. Blood Sugar Regulation:

Individuals with diabetes or insulin resistance need to carefully manage their blood sugar levels. Fasting can have a significant impact on blood sugar, so it's crucial to consult a healthcare provider for guidance.

8. Eating disorders or disordered eating patterns:
Those with a history of eating disorders or unhealthy relationships with food should approach fasting with extreme caution. It may be contraindicated for some individuals.

9. Mental Health and Emotional Well-Being:
Consider your emotional and mental state. Fasting can sometimes affect mood and mental clarity. If you have a history of mental health concerns, consult a mental health professional before fasting.

10. Physical Activity Levels:
Your activity level and exercise routine may need to be adjusted during a fast. It's important to balance physical activity with your body's energy needs.

Always consult with a healthcare provider or registered dietitian before embarking on any significant fasting regimen, especially if you have any health concerns or conditions. They can provide personalized advice and help you make an informed decision about the best approach for your specific situation.

2. Experience and familiarity:If you're new to fasting, you might want to start with a more manageable approach like intermittent fasting before attempting more extended or intensive fasts.

3. Goals and Intentions:Define your objectives for fasting. Are you looking for weight management, improved mental clarity, spiritual or religious reasons, or other specific benefits? Different types of fasting may align better with different goals.

4. Lifestyle and Schedule:Consider your daily routine. Some fasts may be more

practical and easier to integrate into your schedule than others.

5. Hydration Preferences:Some fasts, like water fasting, involve abstaining from all food and drink except water. Others, like juice fasting, allow for some liquid intake. Choose based on your comfort level and hydration needs.

6. Support and Resources:Do you have access to the necessary resources and information for your chosen fast? This includes things like appropriate foods and beverages, supplements, or any additional tools or equipment.

7. Duration of Fast: Decide how long you plan to fast. Some fasts, like intermittent fasting, can be done daily, while others, like water fasting, are typically shorter but more intensive.

8. Personal Preferences:Take into account your personal preferences, tastes, and comfort level with different fasting methods. It's important to choose a course that you feel confident and comfortable undertaking.

9. Consult a professional:If you have any doubts or concerns, it's always wise to consult with a healthcare provider or a registered dietitian. They can offer personalized advice based on your specific health situation.

Remember, there's no one-size-fits-all approach to fasting, and what works for one person may not work for another. It's about finding a fasting method that aligns with your goals, lifestyle, and health considerations.

CHAPTER 5
THE FASTING PROCESS

- Day-to-Day Experience
- Hydration and Nutrition
- Dealing with Hunger and Cravings

The fasting process can vary depending on the type of fast you're undertaking. Here, I'll give a general overview of what you might expect during a typical fast:

1. Beginning the Fast:
You start by abstaining from food and, in some cases, certain beverages. This marks the beginning of the fasting period.

2. Initial Hunger and Adjustment:
In the first few hours, you may experience some hunger pangs or cravings as your body adjusts to the absence of food.

3. The body's energy source:
When you don't consume food, your body begins to rely on stored glycogen for energy. Once glycogen stores are depleted, it turns to fat for fuel.

4. Increased mental clarity:
Some people report feeling mentally clear and focused during a fast as the body shifts into a state of ketosis (burning fat for energy).

5. Hydration is key.
Staying well-hydrated is crucial. Drinking water helps maintain bodily functions and supports overall well-being.

6. Potential Detoxification:
Depending on the fast, there may be a detoxification effect as the body expels waste and toxins.

7. Periods of Weakness or Fatigue:
Especially during extended fasts, you might experience moments of weakness or fatigue.

It's important to rest and listen to your body.

8. Fasting Adaptation:
With time, your body adapts to the fasting state, and hunger signals may diminish.

9. Emotional and Mental States:
Some people experience shifts in mood or emotions during fasting. It's important to practice self-awareness and mindfulness.

10. Breaking the Fast:
When it's time to end the fast, it's crucial to do so gradually and with care. Begin with light, easily digestible foods.

11. Post-Fast Nutrition:
After the fast, it's important to nourish your body with balanced and nutritious meals to replenish energy stores.

12. Reflecting on the Experience:
Take some time to reflect on your fasting experience. Consider what went well and

whether there are any adjustments you'd like to make for future fasts.

Remember, fasting experiences can vary widely from person to person. It's important to listen to your body and make adjustments as needed. If at any point you feel unwell or experience concerning symptoms, it's crucial to seek medical attention promptly. Additionally, consulting a healthcare provider before starting any significant fast is recommended, especially for individuals with underlying health conditions.

The day-to-day experience of fasting can be a unique and individualized journey. It depends on the type of fast you're undertaking, your personal habits, and how your body responds to the changes. Here's a general outline of what you might expect during a typical day of fasting:

1. Pre-Dawn (Suhoor): Morning Meal:
For those observing religious fasting like

Ramadan, this meal is consumed before sunrise. It typically includes complex carbohydrates, protein, healthy fats, and plenty of water to sustain you throughout the day.

2. Daytime Hours:
During the fast, you abstain from food and, depending on the fast, possibly beverages as well. You might experience periods of hunger, especially in the early stages of the fast.

3. Staying Hydrated:
It's crucial to stay well hydrated during a fast. This often involves drinking water in between meals and during non-fasting hours.

4. Midday and Afternoon:
Depending on your body's response to fasting, you may experience fluctuations in energy levels. Some people report increased mental clarity and focus.

5. Preparation for Evening (Iftar): Evening Meal:
For those observing religious fasting, this meal is consumed after sunset. It's a special time for families and communities to come together. The meal typically starts with dates and water, followed by a balanced selection of foods.

6. Breaking the Fast:
Starting with dates and water is a common practice. This is followed by a balanced meal that includes protein, complex carbohydrates, vegetables, and fruits.

7. Evening Activities:
Depending on the type of fast and cultural or religious practices, evenings may involve social and religious activities.

8. Nighttime Rest:
Ensuring you get enough rest is important during a fast to support your body's healing and rejuvenation processes.

9. Mindfulness and Reflection:
Fasting can provide a time for introspection, gratitude, and spiritual reflection, especially in religious fasting practices.

10. Listening to Your Body:
Pay attention to how your body feels throughout the day. If you experience discomfort or unusual symptoms, it's important to address them.

11. Repeat the Cycle:
The next day, you'll wake up to begin the fasting process again.

Remember, everyone's experience with fasting is different. Some may find it empowering and spiritually uplifting, while others may face challenges. It's important to be kind to yourself and to seek support if needed. If you experience any adverse effects during the fast, it's crucial to seek medical attention promptly. Consulting a healthcare provider before starting any significant fast is recommended, especially for individuals with underlying health conditions.

Hydration and nutrition are crucial aspects to consider when fasting. Properly managing your intake of fluids and nutrients can help support your health and well-being during a fast. Here are some guidelines for staying adequately hydrated and nourished:

Hydration:

1. Water Intake:
Drink plenty of water during non-fasting hours. This is especially important for preventing dehydration.

2. Electrolytes:
Consider including electrolyte-rich beverages or supplements, especially if you're fasting for an extended period. This helps maintain a balance of essential

minerals like sodium, potassium, and magnesium.

3. Avoid overconsumption.
While it's important to stay hydrated, avoid excessive drinking of water in a short period of time, as this can lead to a condition called water intoxication or hyponatremia.

4. Monitor Urine Color:
Use the color of your urine as a general indicator of your hydration status. Pale yellow to clear urine is a good sign of adequate hydration.

Nutrition:

1. Balanced Meals:
When you do eat, focus on balanced meals that include a variety of nutrients. Include sources of protein, complex carbohydrates, healthy fats, and plenty of fruits and vegetables.

2. Fiber Intake:
If your fast allows for solid food, choose

foods that are rich in fiber. Fiber helps with satiety and supports digestive health.

3. Avoid excessive sugars.
If consuming juices or sugary beverages, be mindful of the sugar content. Too much sugar can lead to rapid spikes and drops in blood sugar levels.

4. Supplements (if needed):
Depending on the type and duration of your fast, you may need to consider supplements like vitamins or minerals. Consult a healthcare provider for personalized advice.

5. Avoid overindulgence.
When breaking a fast, start with small, easily digestible meals. Overeating can lead to discomfort and digestive issues.

6. Whole Foods:
Whenever possible, choose whole, minimally processed foods. These provide a wide range of essential nutrients and are generally more nourishing.

Remember, it's important to consult a healthcare provider or registered dietitian before starting any significant fast, especially if you have underlying health conditions. They can provide personalized advice on how to manage your hydration and nutrition during the fast and help you make choices that support your well-being.

Managing hunger and cravings during fasting can be challenging, but there are several strategies you can try:

1. Stay hydrated. Drink plenty of water throughout the day. Sometimes thirst can be mistaken for hunger.

2. Choose nutrient-dense foods: When you do eat, focus on foods that are rich in nutrients. This helps keep you satiated for longer.

3. Include fiber and protein: fiber-rich foods (like fruits, vegetables, and whole grains) and protein (such as lean meats, legumes, and nuts) can help you feel full.

4. Plan balanced meals: If you're breaking your fast, aim for a balanced meal with a mix of carbohydrates, protein, and healthy fats. This can help stabilize blood sugar levels.

5. Avoid sugary foods and drinks: They can lead to rapid spikes and drops in blood sugar, which can increase cravings.

6. Incorporate healthy fats: avocados, nuts, and olive oil can help provide a sense of fullness.

7. Chew gum or drink herbal tea: These can provide a distraction and curb cravings.

8. Practice mindful eating: pay attention to your hunger cues and eat slowly. This can help prevent overeating.

9. Keep Busy: Engage in activities that occupy your mind and keep you from thinking about food.

10. Listen to your body: If you're genuinely hungry, it's okay to eat. It's important to prioritize your health and well-being.

11. Consider Your Fasting Schedule: Adjust your fasting window if needed. It's important to find a routine that works for your body and lifestyle.

Remember, it's crucial to consult a healthcare professional or registered dietitian before making significant changes to your diet, especially if you have underlying health conditions. They can provide personalized advice tailored to your needs.

CHAPTER 6.
BREAKING YOUR FAST

- Transitioning Back to Regular Eating
- Post-Fast Nutrition

Breaking a fast is an important step, and it's crucial to do it in a way that is gentle on your digestive system. Here are some tips:

1. Start with Water: Begin by rehydrating yourself with a glass of water. This helps kickstart your digestive system.

2. Opt for nutrient-dense foods: Begin with foods that are easy on the stomach and provide essential nutrients. Consider fruits, vegetables, lean proteins, or whole grains.

3. Avoid heavy or gritty foods. Steer clear of fried or overly processed foods, as they can be harder to digest after a period of fasting.

4. Go Slow and Small: Start with small portions to allow your digestive system to adjust. Eating too quickly or too much can lead to discomfort.

5. Chew thoroughly: Properly chewing your food aids in digestion and can help prevent digestive issues.

6. Include Protein and Fiber: These nutrients can help stabilize your blood sugar levels and keep you feeling satisfied.

7. Avoid sugary foods. While they might provide a quick energy boost, sugary foods can lead to a spike in blood sugar levels followed by a crash.

8. Listen to Your Body: Pay attention to how you feel as you eat. Stop when you're comfortably full.

9. Consider bone broth or light soups: These can be gentle on your digestive system while providing essential nutrients.

10. Wait Before Introducing Heavy Foods: If you're transitioning from a longer fast, it's a good idea to wait a bit before introducing more complex or heavy meals.

Every person's body is different, so it's important to pay attention to how you feel and adjust your approach accordingly. If you experience any discomfort or unusual symptoms while breaking your fast, it's best to consult a healthcare professional.

Transitioning back to regular eating after a fast is an important process to ensure your body adjusts smoothly. Start with easily digestible foods like fruits and vegetables, and gradually introduce lean proteins and whole grains. It's crucial to listen to your body's hunger cues and eat until you're satisfied, rather than overindulging. Staying hydrated is also key. Remember, consulting a healthcare professional for personalized advice is recommended, especially if you're considering longer or more intensive fasts.

Post-Fast Nutrition

After a period of fasting, it's crucial to reintroduce food thoughtfully and gradually. Begin with easily digestible options like fruits, vegetables, and smoothies to gently awaken your digestive system. Hydration is paramount; opt for water, herbal teas, or electrolyte-rich fluids.

As the day progresses, incorporate lean proteins like poultry, fish, or plant-based sources, along with complex carbohydrates such as whole grains. Include healthy fats like avocados, nuts, and olive oil for sustained energy.

Listen to your body's signals of hunger and fullness, and avoid excessive or processed foods. Focus on nutrient-dense choices to support your body's recovery.

Remember, individual needs may vary, so consulting a healthcare professional or dietitian for personalized guidance is always a wise step.

CHAPTER 7

MONITORING PROGRESS AND LISTENING TO YOUR BODY

- Tracking Physical Changes
- Understanding Signals from Your Body

Monitoring your progress during fasting is crucial for a safe and effective experience. Here are some key points to keep in mind:

1. Regular check-ins: Take time to assess how you're feeling throughout your fast. Pay attention to any physical or emotional changes.

2. Listen to Your Body: Your body will give you signals about its needs. If you experience severe discomfort, dizziness, or weakness, it's important to reevaluate your fasting approach.

3. Hydration: Ensure you're adequately hydrating yourself. Drink water and

electrolyte-rich beverages to maintain proper bodily functions.

4. Keep Track of Time: Note the start and end times of your fasts. This helps establish a routine and enables you to track your progress over time.

5. Energy Levels: Observe your energy levels. If you notice a significant drop in energy, consider adjusting the duration or type of fasting you're undertaking.

6. Physical Measurements: If weight management is a goal, you may choose to monitor your weight or take body measurements periodically. However, remember that this is just one aspect of progress.

7. Mental and Emotional Well-Being: Pay attention to your mood and mental clarity. Fasting can affect cognitive functions, so it's important to be mindful of any changes.

8. Journaling: Keep a journal to record your experiences, feelings, and any insights gained during your fasting journey. This can be a valuable tool for reflection.

9. Consult a professional: If you have any medical conditions or concerns, seek advice from a healthcare professional. They can offer guidance tailored to your individual health circumstances.

10. Adapt as Needed: Be flexible in your approach. If you encounter challenges or your body reacts in unexpected ways, don't hesitate to modify your fasting routine.

Don't forget, fasting is a personal practice, and what works best for one person may not be suitable for another. Trust your instincts and prioritize your well-being above all else.

Tracking physical changes during fasting can provide valuable insights into your body's response to this practice. Here are some key aspects to consider:

1. Weight: Monitor changes in your weight. Keep in mind that weight fluctuations can occur due to various factors, including water retention, so focus on long-term trends rather than day-to-day variations.

2. Body Measurements: Take measurements of specific areas like the waist, hips, chest, and limbs. This can provide a more comprehensive view of changes in body composition.

3. Body Fat Percentage: Consider using methods like skinfold calipers, bioelectrical impedance scales, or DEXA scans to measure body fat percentage. This offers a more accurate assessment of changes in body composition.

4. Muscle Mass: Track changes in muscle mass. Maintaining or increasing muscle mass is important for overall health and metabolism.

5. Energy Levels: Note any changes in your energy levels. Increased energy may be a positive sign, while a significant drop may indicate a need for adjustment in your fasting regimen.

6. Physical Performance: If you engage in regular physical activity or exercise, monitor your performance. Pay attention to any improvements or declines in strength, endurance, and flexibility.

7. Appearance of Skin and Hair: Observe any changes in the condition of your skin and hair. Some individuals may notice improvements in skin complexion and hair health during fasting.

8. Digestive Health: Take note of any changes in digestive function. Some people experience improvements in digestion and reduced bloating during fasting.

9. Water Retention: Be aware of fluctuations in water retention, which can affect weight and body measurements. This is normal and

may not necessarily indicate a significant physical change.

10. Consult a Professional: If you have specific health goals or concerns, consider seeking guidance from a healthcare professional or a registered dietitian. They can provide personalized advice and help interpret the physical changes you observe.

Remember to approach tracking with a balanced perspective. While it can be informative, it's important not to obsess over the numbers. Focus on how you feel overall and prioritize your well-being throughout the fasting process.

Understanding Signals from your body during fasting

Understanding the signals your body sends during fasting is crucial for a safe and beneficial fasting experience. Here's a breakdown of key signals and what they may mean:

1. Hunger Pangs: Mild feelings of hunger are normal during fasting. It's a sign that your body is using stored energy. However, severe or prolonged hunger may indicate a need to reevaluate your fasting approach.

2. Dehydration can lead to feelings of thirst. Stay well-hydrated by drinking water, herbal teas, and electrolyte-rich beverages. Pay attention to your body's signals for thirst.

3. Weakness or dizziness: These sensations can indicate low blood sugar or dehydration. If you experience severe weakness or dizziness, it may be a sign to break your fast and seek nourishment.

4. Increased Mental Clarity: Some individuals experience enhanced mental clarity and focus during fasting. This can be a positive signal, indicating that your body is adapting well to the fasting regimen.

5. Fatigue: Fasting can lead to reduced energy levels, especially if your body is not yet accustomed to the practice. Adequate rest and proper nutrition after breaking your fast can help alleviate fatigue.

6. Digestive Changes: Pay attention to how your digestive system reacts. Some people may experience improved digestion, while others may need to make adjustments to their fasting routine to avoid discomfort.

7. Mood and Emotional Changes: Fasting can impact your mood and emotional well-being. Some may feel a sense of clarity and calm, while others may experience mood swings. It's important to be mindful of these changes.

8. Headaches: Mild headaches can occur due to factors like dehydration or changes in blood sugar levels. If headaches persist or worsen, it may be a sign to reevaluate your fasting regimen.

9. Increased Satiety: Over time, you may notice that you feel more satiated with smaller portions of food. This is a positive signal that your body is becoming more efficient at utilizing nutrients.

10. Cravings: Pay attention to any cravings you experience. Understanding your cravings can help you make informed choices about the types of foods you consume when breaking your fast.

11. Consult a professional: If you experience severe or persistent discomfort or if you have underlying health concerns, consult a healthcare professional. They can provide personalized advice based on your individual circumstances.

Remember that everyone is different, and what works for one person may not work for another. Listening to your body and being attuned to its signals is key to a safe and beneficial fasting experience.

CHAPTER 8.

POTENTIAL RISKS AND SAFETY CONSIDERATIONS

- Common Mistakes to Avoid
- When to Seek Professional Advice

Avoiding common mistakes in fasting can help ensure a safe and effective experience. Here are some key pitfalls to be mindful of:

1. Skipping Hydration: Failing to drink enough water can lead to dehydration. Stay well hydrated by consuming water, herbal teas, and electrolyte-rich beverages.

2. Ignoring Hunger Signals: Ignoring severe or prolonged hunger pangs can be detrimental to your health. It's important to listen to your body and consider breaking your fast if necessary.

3. Overcompensating After Fasting: Binge-eating or consuming excessive amounts of unhealthy foods when breaking your fast can negate the benefits of fasting. Opt for nutritious, balanced meals.

4. Neglecting Nutrient Intake: Fasting doesn't mean neglecting essential nutrients. Ensure you're still getting a variety of vitamins, minerals, and macronutrients during your eating window.

5. Overestimating abilities: Starting with overly ambitious fasting schedules can lead to physical discomfort or fatigue. Begin with shorter fasts and gradually extend them as your body adapts.

6. Ignoring Medical Advice: If you have underlying health conditions or are on medication, it's crucial to consult a healthcare professional before starting a fasting regimen.

7. Lack of Rest and Sleep: Adequate rest is important during fasting. Avoid overexertion and prioritize getting enough sleep to support your body's functions.

8. Neglecting Electrolytes: Alongside water, electrolytes like sodium, potassium, and magnesium are essential for proper bodily function. Consider including electrolyte-rich foods or supplements.

9. Fasting for the Wrong Reasons: Fasting should be approached with clear intentions. Using fasting solely as a means for rapid weight loss or extreme calorie restriction may not yield sustainable results.

10. Ignoring Emotional Well-Being: Fasting can affect your mood and emotions. Be mindful of these changes and practice self-care to support your mental health.

11. Fasting Without Flexibility: Being overly rigid in your fasting schedule can lead to

stress and discomfort. It's important to be flexible and adjust your fasting routine as needed.

12. Not Breaking Fast Mindfully: Breaking your fast with heavy, processed, or sugary foods can lead to digestive discomfort. Opt for nutrient-dense, easily digestible options.

13. Comparing Yourself to Others: Each person's body responds differently to fasting. Avoid comparing your progress or experiences to others, and focus on your own well-being.

Remember, fasting is a personal journey, and it's crucial to prioritize your health and well-being throughout the process. If in doubt, seek guidance from a healthcare professional or a registered dietitian.

Seeking professional advice during fasting is important, especially if you have specific health concerns or medical conditions. Here are situations in which it's advisable to consult a healthcare professional or a registered dietitian:

1. Underlying Health Conditions: If you have any pre-existing medical conditions such as diabetes, heart disease, kidney problems, or gastrointestinal issues, it's crucial to consult a healthcare provider before starting a fasting regimen.

2. Medication Use: If you are taking medications, especially those that need to be taken with food or at specific times, seek advice from a healthcare professional to ensure that fasting won't interfere with your medication schedule.

3. Pregnancy or Breastfeeding: Fasting during pregnancy or while breastfeeding can have significant impacts on both maternal and fetal health. It's essential to get specialized advice from a healthcare provider.

4. Eating Disorders or History of Disordered Eating: Individuals with a history of eating disorders or disordered eating patterns should approach fasting with caution and under the guidance of a healthcare professional.

5. Severe or Prolonged Discomfort: If you experience severe or prolonged discomfort during fasting, such as extreme dizziness, weakness, chest pain, or other concerning symptoms, seek immediate medical attention.

6. Unintended Weight Loss: If you're losing weight rapidly and it's not part of your intended fasting goal, or if you're experiencing unintended changes in appetite, it's important to consult a healthcare provider.

7. Excessive Fatigue or Lethargy: Persistent fatigue or a significant drop in energy levels may indicate that your body is not adapting

well to the fasting regimen. Seek professional advice to address this.

8. Changes in Mental Health: If fasting is causing significant changes in your mood, behavior, or mental well-being, it's important to discuss this with a healthcare professional.

9. Irregular Menstrual Cycles: For individuals with menstrual cycles, irregularities or disruptions may occur with fasting. Seek advice if you notice changes in your menstrual patterns.

10. Children and adolescents: Fasting in children and adolescents requires special consideration due to their growing and developing bodies. Consult a pediatrician or healthcare professional before implementing any fasting regimen.

11. Long-Term or Extended Fasting: Extended fasts, typically lasting more than 24–48 hours, can carry additional risks and

should only be undertaken under the supervision of a healthcare professional.

Always remember that your health and well-being should be your top priorities. If you have any doubts or concerns about fasting, seeking advice from a healthcare professional or registered dietitian is a prudent step. They can provide personalized guidance based on your individual health circumstances.

CHAPTER 9

COMBINING FASTING WITH A HEALTHY LIFESTYLE

- Exercise and Physical Activity
- Balanced Nutrition

Engaging in exercise and physical activity during fasting requires careful consideration to ensure your body's needs are met. Here are some tips to keep in mind:

1. Low-Intensity Activities: Light activities like walking, stretching, or gentle yoga can be beneficial during fasting. They help maintain mobility and can be performed without excessive strain.

2. Avoid strenuous workouts: high-intensity workouts, heavy weightlifting, or intense cardio can lead to increased fatigue and may not be advisable during fasting, especially for extended periods.

3. Timing Matters: If you choose to exercise, consider doing so during non-fasting periods or right before you break your fast. This allows you to replenish energy and nutrients post-workout.

4. Listen to Your Body: Pay close attention to how you feel. If you experience dizziness, weakness, or extreme fatigue, it's important to stop exercising and rest.

5. Stay Hydrated: Proper hydration is crucial, especially when combining exercise with fasting. Drink water and electrolyte-rich beverages to prevent dehydration.

6. Balanced Nutrition After Exercise: When you do break your fast after exercising, prioritize nutrient-dense foods that replenish energy and support muscle recovery.

7. Modify Intensity and Duration: If you're used to intense workouts, consider scaling down the intensity and duration during fasting. Focus on maintaining activity rather than pushing yourself to your limits.

8. Warm-Up and Cool-Down: Ensure you incorporate proper warm-up and cool-down routines to reduce the risk of injury and allow your body to adjust to exercise.

9. Be Mindful of Overexertion: Pushing yourself too hard during fasting can lead to overexertion, which may have negative effects on your health. It's better to prioritize gentle, moderate exercise.

Don't forget, the goal is to support your body's well-being, not to strain it unnecessarily. Always prioritize safety and listen to your body's signals. If in doubt, it's best to choose lighter, low-impact activities during fasting.

Combining fasting with balanced nutrition is essential for a safe and effective fasting experience. Here are some tips to achieve this balance:

1. Diversify Your Diet: Ensure your meals include a variety of food groups like fruits, vegetables, whole grains, lean proteins, and healthy fats to provide a wide range of nutrients.

2. Prioritize Whole Foods: Choose minimally processed, whole foods over highly processed options. This includes fresh fruits and vegetables, whole grains, nuts, seeds, and lean proteins.

3. Include lean proteins: Incorporate lean sources of protein like poultry, fish, tofu, legumes, and low-fat dairy. Protein helps with satiety and supports muscle health.

4. Fiber-Rich Foods: Opt for high-fiber options like whole grains, fruits, and vegetables. Fiber aids digestion and helps keep you feeling full.

5. Healthy Fats: Include sources of healthy fats such as avocados, nuts, seeds, and olive oil. These provide essential fatty acids and help keep you satisfied.

6. Control Portion Sizes: Pay attention to portion sizes to avoid overeating. Fasting can sometimes lead to larger meals, so being mindful of portion control is important.

7. Stay Hydrated: Drink plenty of water and consider incorporating hydrating foods like fruits and vegetables into your meals.

8. Balanced Macronutrients: Aim for a balanced distribution of carbohydrates, proteins, and fats in your meals to provide sustained energy throughout the fasting period.

9. Plan nutrient-dense snacks: If your eating window is limited, have nutritious snacks available to ensure you meet your nutrient needs. This could include nuts, seeds, yogurt, or whole fruits.

10. Avoid Sugary and Processed Foods: Minimize or avoid foods high in added sugars, refined carbohydrates, and processed snacks. These can lead to rapid spikes and drops in blood sugar levels.

11. Supplement wisely: If you have specific nutrient needs, consult a healthcare professional or registered dietitian for guidance on supplements that may complement your fasting regimen.

12. Mindful Eating: Take time to savor your meals. Eating slowly and mindfully can help you recognize when you're full and prevent overeating.

Remember, the key is to nourish your body in a way that supports your health and well-being, whether you're in a fasting or eating period. A balanced and nutrient-rich diet can help you make the most of your fasting experience.

CHAPTER 10
LONG-TERM FASTING AND MAINTENANCE

- Incorporating Fasting into Your Routine
- Sustainable Practices

Integrating fasting into your routine can be done in a mindful and balanced way. Here's a suggestion for incorporating intermittent fasting, a popular approach:

1. Choose a fasting window:

Decide on a daily fasting window. A common option is the 16/8 method (16 hours of fasting, 8 hours of eating).

2. Select Your Eating Window:

Plan when you'll eat during the 8-hour window. This can vary based on your schedule and preferences. For example, 12:00 PM–8:00 PM or 1:00 PM–9:00 PM

3. Gradual Adjustment:

If you're new to fasting, ease into it by gradually increasing your fasting window over a week or two.

4. Stay Hydrated:

Drink water, herbal teas, or black coffee during the fasting period to stay hydrated.

5. Balanced Meals:

Ensure your meals are well-balanced with a mix of lean protein, healthy fats, complex carbohydrates, and plenty of fruits and vegetables.

6. Listen to your body:

Pay attention to your hunger cues. If you feel excessively hungry or ill, it's okay to break your fast earlier.

7. Adjust based on activity level:

On more active days, you might need to adjust your fasting window or consume more calories within it.

8. Monitor nutrient intake:

Be mindful of getting enough essential nutrients. Consider consulting a healthcare professional or nutritionist for guidance.

9. Exercise Considerations:

You can engage in light to moderate exercise during the fasting period, but consider scheduling intense workouts within your eating window.

10. Flexibility:

Don't be afraid to adjust your fasting routine as needed. It's important to make it sustainable for your lifestyle and well-being.

Remember, fasting isn't suitable for everyone. It's crucial to consult a healthcare professional, especially if you have any underlying health conditions or concerns.

They can provide personalized advice and monitor your progress.

Sustainable practices

Sustainable fasting practices aim to promote both physical and environmental well-being. Here are some approaches:

1. Intermittent Fasting: This involves cycling between periods of eating and fasting. It can help improve metabolic health and reduce food waste.

2. Seasonal Fasting: Eating foods that are in-season can reduce the need for transportation and refrigeration, lowering carbon emissions.

3. Plant-Based Fasting: Choosing plant-based foods during fasts can reduce the environmental impact associated with animal agriculture.

4. Mindful Eating: Being conscious of portion sizes and reducing food waste helps conserve resources.

5. Water Fasting: For short durations, water-only fasts can promote detoxification and reduce consumption of processed foods.

6. Zero-Waste Fasting: Opt for package-free, whole foods to minimize packaging waste.

7. Community Fasts: Organize group fasts to build a sense of community and support sustainable practices.

8. Energy Conservation: During fasting hours, minimize electricity and water usage to further reduce your environmental footprint.

it's important to consult with a healthcare professional before making significant changes to your diet or fasting practices. They can provide personalized advice based on your individual health needs.

CHAPTER 11.

FASTING AND MENTAL WELL-BEING

- Mindfulness and Meditation
- Fasting and Mental Clarity

-Mindfulness and Meditation

Practicing mindfulness and meditation can be beneficial during fasting. They can help you stay focused, reduce stress, and maintain a sense of calm. When incorporating them into your fasting routine, consider the following tips:

1. Set an intention: Begin your meditation with a clear intention related to your fasting. This could be to cultivate self-discipline, connect with your body's signals, or find inner strength.

2. Focus on Breath Awareness: Pay attention to your breath. Deep, slow breaths can help you relax and maintain a sense of presence.

3. Body Scan Meditation: Conduct a body scan to bring awareness to different parts of your body. This can help you notice any areas of tension or discomfort and promote relaxation.

4. Mindful Eating: When you do break your fast, practice mindful eating. Pay attention to the tastes, textures, and sensations of the food. This can enhance your appreciation for nourishment.

5. Observe Hunger Signals: Mindfulness can help you discern genuine hunger from cravings or emotional cues. This awareness can guide you to make mindful choices when you decide to eat.

6. Practice gratitude: reflect on the privilege of having access to food and the ability to fast. This sense of gratitude can deepen your connection to the experience.

7. Use guided meditations: There are various guided meditations specifically designed for fasting. They often incorporate affirmations and visualizations to support your fasting journey.

Mindfulness and meditation are personal practices, so feel free to adapt them to suit your needs and preferences. Always listen to your body and adjust your fasting schedule accordingly. If you have any underlying health conditions, consult a healthcare professional before making significant changes to your fasting routine.

- Fasting and Mental Clarity

Fasting can potentially have an impact on mental clarity, though individual experiences may vary. Here's how fasting may influence mental clarity:

1. Stabilizing Blood Sugar: Fasting can lead to more stable blood sugar levels. This can

prevent spikes and crashes, which are associated with mental fog and fatigue.

2. Enhancing Brain-Derived Neurotrophic Factor (BDNF): Some studies suggest that fasting may increase the production of BDNF, a protein that supports the growth and survival of neurons. This could potentially improve cognitive function.

3. Ketosis and Cognitive Function: Extended fasting or very low-carb diets can lead to a state of ketosis, where the body uses ketones for energy. Some people report increased mental clarity and focus during ketosis.

4. Reducing Inflammation: Fasting may help reduce inflammation, which can have positive effects on brain health. Chronic inflammation has been linked to cognitive decline.

5. Improved Sleep: For some individuals, fasting may lead to improved sleep quality. Better sleep can contribute to enhanced cognitive function and mental clarity.

6. Psychological Benefits: Fasting rituals can have psychological benefits, promoting a sense of discipline, focus, and mindfulness, which can indirectly contribute to mental clarity.

7. Caution with Prolonged Fasting: While short-term fasting may have cognitive benefits for some individuals, prolonged or extreme fasting can lead to nutrient deficiencies and negatively impact mental function.

It's important to approach fasting with caution and consider individual factors like overall health, nutritional needs, and any existing medical conditions. Always consult a healthcare professional before making significant changes to your fasting routine, especially if you have concerns about its impact on your mental well-being. Additionally, listen to your body and adjust your fasting schedule as needed to ensure it aligns with your overall well-being.

Conclusion

Embarking on a fasting journey can be a profound and transformative experience. It requires discipline, mindfulness, and a deep understanding of one's body and its needs. Throughout this journey, individuals often encounter a range of physical and mental shifts:

1. Increased Awareness of Eating Habits:
Fasting prompts a closer examination of our relationship with food. It highlights emotional triggers, habitual eating patterns, and the importance of mindful consumption.

2. Heightened Appreciation for Nourishment:
Breaking a fast can bring about a newfound appreciation for the flavors and textures of food. Every meal becomes a moment of gratitude for sustenance.

3. Improved Physical Health:
Many experience positive changes such as weight loss, stabilized blood sugar levels, reduced inflammation, and enhanced metabolic function. These improvements can lead to a sense of vitality and well-being.

4. Enhanced Mental Clarity:
Fasting can clear the mental fog and bring about a sense of mental sharpness and focus. This clarity often leads to increased productivity and a heightened sense of mental acuity.

5. Deeper Connection with Body Signals:
Learning to differentiate between true hunger and cravings becomes a crucial skill. Fasters often develop a heightened sensitivity to their bodies signals for nourishment.

6. Emotional Resilience and Discipline:
Successfully completing a fast requires a level of discipline and self-control. This can translate into increased resilience when

facing challenges both within and outside of the fasting journey.

7. Potential for Spiritual or Reflective Insights:
For some, fasting can be a deeply spiritual experience, providing an opportunity for introspection, meditation, and a heightened sense of connection with oneself or a higher power.

8. Balanced Approach to Nutrition:
Fasting can encourage a more balanced and intentional approach to nutrition. It prompts consideration of the quality and composition of the foods we consume.

It's important to remember that fasting is a highly individual practice. What works for one person may not work for another, and it's crucial to approach any fasting regimen with awareness, education, and consideration for one's unique health circumstances.

Before beginning any significant dietary changes, especially fasting, it's advisable to consult a healthcare professional or registered dietitian to ensure they align with your specific health needs and goals.

www.ingramcontent.com/pod-product-compliance
Lightning Source LLC
Chambersburg PA
CBHW061000260726
48661CB00005B/1968